Mediter

CW01560593

Diet

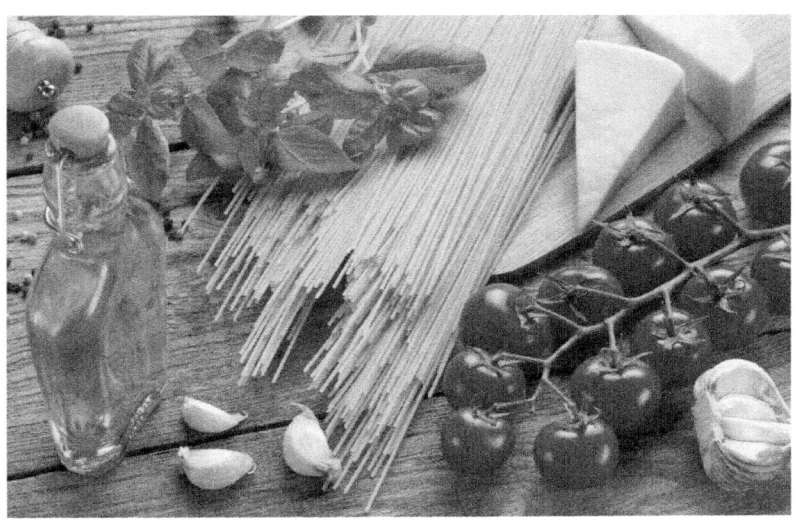

A Complete Beginners Guide to Lose Weight and

Feel your best eating delicious food

Sofia Lewis

ISBN: 1523633239

ISBN-13: 978-1523633234

DEDICATION

I dedicate this book to all the people who have a love for delicious food and for the beautiful Mediterranean culture and food.

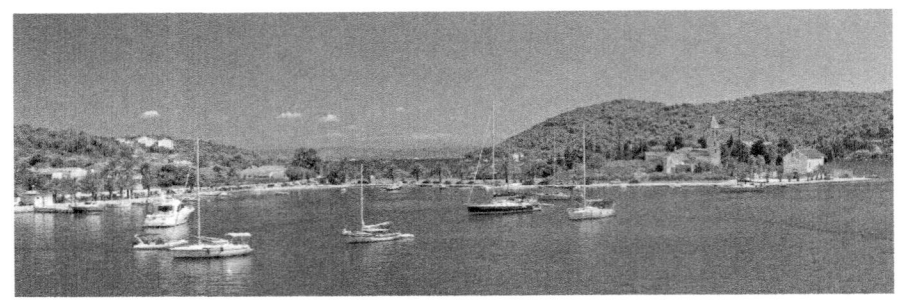

CONTENTS

DISCLAIMER

This document is geared towards providing exact and reliable information in regards to the topic and issue covered. The publication is sold with the idea that the publisher is not required to render accounting, officially permitted, or otherwise, qualified services. If advice is necessary, legal or professional, a practiced individual in the profession should be ordered.

- From a Declaration of Principles which was accepted and approved equally by a Committee of the American Bar Association and a Committee of Publishers and Associations.

The information provided herein is stated to be truthful and consistent, in that any liability, in terms of inattention or otherwise, by any usage or abuse of any policies, processes, or directions contained within is the solitary and utter responsibility of the recipient reader. Under no circumstances will any legal responsibility or blame be held against the publisher for any reparation, damages, or monetary loss due to the information herein, either directly or indirectly.

Respective authors own all copyrights not held by the publisher.

The information herein is offered for informational purposes solely, and is universal as so. The presentation of the information is without contract or any type of guarantee assurance.

The trademarks that are used are without any consent, and the publication of the trademark is without permission or backing by the trademark owner. All trademarks and brands within this book are for clarifying purposes only and are the owned by the owners themselves, not affiliated with this document.

.

INTRODUCTION

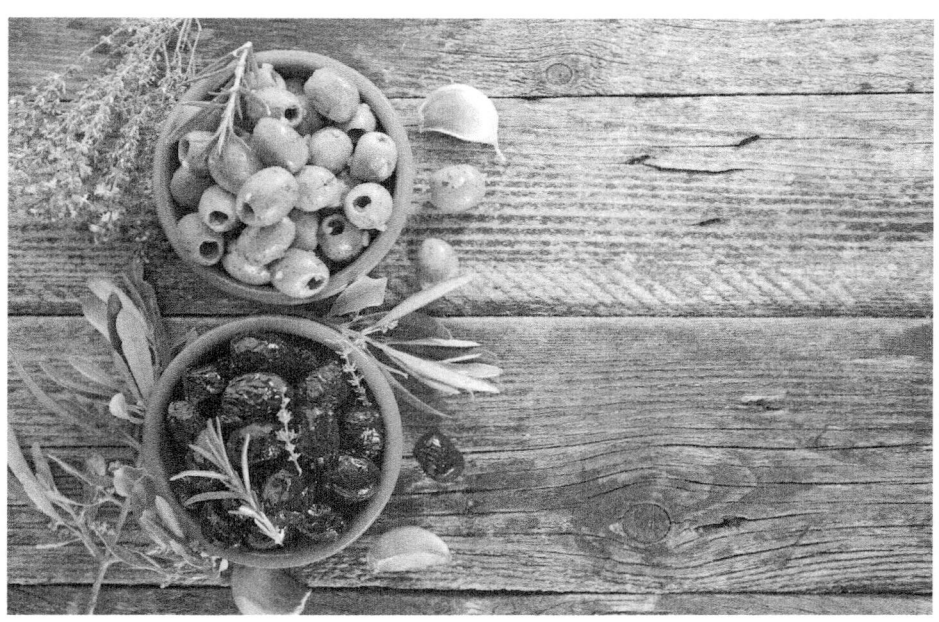

Sixteen countries border the Mediterranean Sea, and as a whole these people have fewer chronic health problems than the rest of the world.

When scientists look at their lifestyle, they find that people in each of these countries live a very similar lifestyle. First, they find that the people eat a variety of foods focusing on fruits, vegetables, nuts beans, seeds, cereals and breads. As many of these foods are seasonal as possible. Secondly, they use olive oil when cooking and when making dressings. Third, they eat a lot of fish, but very little meat. They also eat a moderate amount of cheese and yogurt. They also drink a glass of red wine each day with their meals. A secret to this diet is that the people live a very active lifestyle.

Husband and wife team, Ancel and Margaret Keys, first introduced the Mediterranean diet. It did not enjoy much success until Doctor Walter Willett of Harvard University's School of Public Health and others started recommending the diet. It is based on the wonderful foods that he found in the Crete, Greece, area where the incidence of heart disease was extremely low. The diet focuses on the use of olive oil, unrefined cereals, fruits, vegetables, and legumes. Additionally, dieters are expected to eat a larger amount of fish than many people are currently consuming. Those following the diet drink one glass of red wine each day. The diet also encourages moderate consumption of cheese and yogurt, and eliminates most meat.

Almost no one will go hungry on this diet, as people are encouraged to eat six to 12 servings of fruits and vegetables, four to six servings of grain products, one to three servings of dairy products, one to two servings of poultry or fish each day, along with drinking a glass of red wine.

Dieters can enjoy a vast amount of dishes on this diet, and there is lots of evidence that it works. One of the earliest studies, which was published in 2008 in the peer-reviewed British Medical Journal found that people who strictly followed this diet had a nine percent less chance of dying from any cause. In particular, those following this diet had a nine percent less chance of dying from cardiovascular problems, and a six percent less chance of dying from cancer. Additionally, it was found that individuals following the diet had a 13 percent less chance of developing Alzheimer's and Parkinson diseases. These same findings were also found in an independent study that was published in the American Journal of Clinical Nutrition published in 2010.

A year later, a study published in the Journal of the American College of Cardiology looked at a number of studies to analyze results from 535,000 people following this study. They found that people following the diet had lower blood pressure, lower blood sugar and lower triglycerides.

New research, published in 2014, published in Public Health Nutrition and on PubMed, supports the earlier finding and also found that people following the diet had less chance of developing type 2 diabetes.

The diet is based on traditional Greece diets, and according to a study published in the New England Journal of Medicine, the closer a person stuck to the traditional diet, the longer that they could expect to live. This study points out that when following this diet, it is vital to keep three different factors in mind. First, it is all the different ingredients in the diet that makes it extremely healthy. Secondly, those living in this region have a more relaxed attitude toward eating. They also get plenty of sunshine and physical activity.

WHY HOME-COOKED MEALS ARE HEALTHIER AND CHEAPER

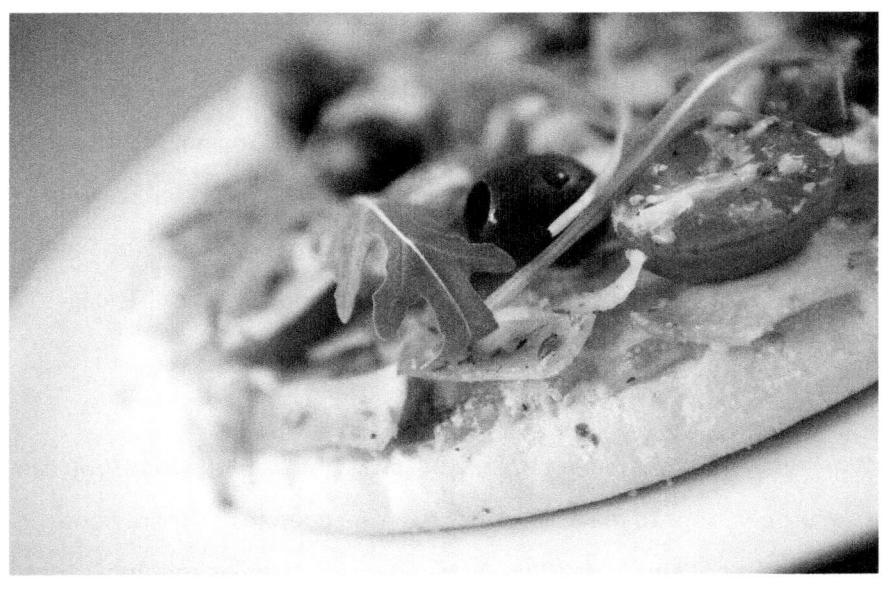

There are many reasons that cooking at home is healthier and cheaper than eating out. Understanding these reasons helps you to live a healthier lifestyle.

When you prepare a meal at home, you know what is in the food. Take the case of David Scheiding who stopped for a sandwich at a popular fast food restaurant. While eating the sandwich, David found a piece of human skin in the sandwich. It turns out that while the manager was dicing the lettuce earlier in the day that he had sliced his thumb quite badly. While the manager sanitized his thumb and applied a bandage, he did not throw away the lettuce that ended up on David's sandwich. He later sued for $50,000 in court.

One might also want to consider the case of Lauren Coleman, a broke college student who stopped at a popular fast-food restaurant for some fries. Leaving with her fries, she later discovered a bloody bandage in the fries. She returned to the restaurant who offered her a refund and some new fries. An employee even admitted that it was her bandage.

When you prepare food at home, you know what is in the food. You can take proper steps to make sure that the food contains no ingredients that you do not know are there. You know how clean everything is that you use to prepare the food. Additionally, you can prepare the food with the seasonings that you want to use, so it tastes the way that you want it to taste.

Cooking at home is much cheaper than eating a nutritious meal out. The typical fast food meal for a family of four costs about $24, while the typical meal prepared at home for a family of four costs just $14. Imagine the amount of money that you can save even over the course of a month. Three meals a day means you save $30 a day multiplied by 30 days in a month and you have saved $900 a month. That may be enough to pay your mortgage or make your car payment.

People who eat at home consume fewer calories. No, the food is not that bad. In fact, it usually tastes better than the food purchased at a restaurant. Instead, the key lies in eating reasonable servings at home. Amazingly, this even includes when the same foods are prepared, according to Colorado State University. They say that the average grilled chicken in a restaurant has 766 calories, while the average grilled chicken prepared at home has just 434 calories. They also say that the average restaurant lasagna contains 650 calories, while the average lasagna prepared at home has just 340 calories. That is a savings of about 300 calories per main entrée. Additionally, people who eat out are often tempted with bread baskets that contain large amounts of calories, all-you-can-eat buffets, and unlimited high calorie drinks.

Amazingly, research from John Hopkins University found that people who eat at home more than five nights a week even eat fewer calories when they do decide to eat out. Adults who admitted that they cooked at home one time a week or less consumed an average of 2,301 total calories, 84 grams of fat and 135 grams of sugar, while those who cooked at home consumed 2,164 calories, 81 grams of fat and 119 grams of sugar on a daily basis.

There's a reason that many restaurant meals taste so good. It is the amount of fat in the food. While fat gives many dishes the flavor, it is also easy to add flavor to food n so many different ways like using spices. Once you start experimenting, you will discover that you love the taste of food and will not even miss the fat.

When you cook at home, you actually burn calories. Research shows that cooking burns about 139 calories per hour while hand washing dishes burns about 151 calories per hour.

It is easier to connect with the family when people eat at home. Research from Michigan State University shows that teens who regularly eat at home score higher on SAT tests, have fewer behavior problems at school and are more apt to go to college. Additionally, people who eat at home usually enjoy a more stable family life, because sitting around the table gives family members the chance to connect with each other. You can sit at the table as long as you want to without feeling guilty about someone waiting for your table or having to tip the wait staff extra because of how long you took. Other research shows that children who eat at home regularly are 42 percent less likely to drink, 50 percent less likely to smoke and 66 percent less likely to use marijuana.

Eating at home is usually faster than going to a restaurant. Again, according to a study published by Colorado State University, a family spends an average of 83 minutes getting ready to eat, including going to the restaurant, before the food arrives. When eating at home, many meals can be prepared in under 30 minutes.

Eating at home is much better for the environment. According to David Pimentel at the College of Agriculture and Life Sciences of Cornell University, it takes a restaurant seven kilocalories of energy to produce a typical meal. It also requires 10 kilocalories of energy to get the food to the restaurant for a total of 17 kilocalories. Alternatively, the average meal at home requires just nine kilocalories. Therefore, your children and grandchildren will live in a healthier world.

When cooking at home, it is very easy to choose the quality of the ingredients that you put in a dish. For example, if you go grocery shopping and all the bananas are black, then you can simply choose a different fruit to eat. Additionally, there are numerous ways to increase the quality of the food by using range-free eggs, buying organic fruits and vegetables and using the freshest ingredients available.

When you prepare meals where the whole family helps, you are giving children the skills that they need for the rest of their lives. So many people do not know how to cook, so this can be a real advantage. Additionally, you have the chance to influence the way that they think about different ingredients. You also get to enjoy spending quality time together building memories that will last the rest of their lives.

Many people find that they return to the same restaurants every day or at least want to eat the same foods each day. Scientists at the Academy of Nutrition and Dietetics have found that stopping on these cravings may not be based on your willpower, but instead are based on your body's need for certain nutrients. If you find that you are always craving red meat, then make sure that you eat foods that are high in iron. That is why it is essential that the person following the Mediterranean diet eat plenty of legumes, beans, nuts, seeds and dried fruit. Alternatively, if you find yourself craving pizza, then you may not have enough Omega 3 fatty acids in your diet. If this is the case, then eat more fish along with free-range chicken. If you are craving chocolate, then make sure to eat plenty of foods that are high in magnesium like pumpkin seeds, sunflower seeds, cashews, almonds and wheat. If you find that you want foods loaded with sugar and salt, then resist the temptation by eating oysters, nuts, and make sure you are eating enough calcium.

There are so many different reasons to cook at home. The food prepared there is healthier than the food brought in a restaurant. It is also a great way to control portion sizes, along with the taste of the food. Most importantly, it allows you to create a fun family environment building memories that people will remember for the rest of their lives.

WHAT'S THE MEDITERRANEAN DIET?

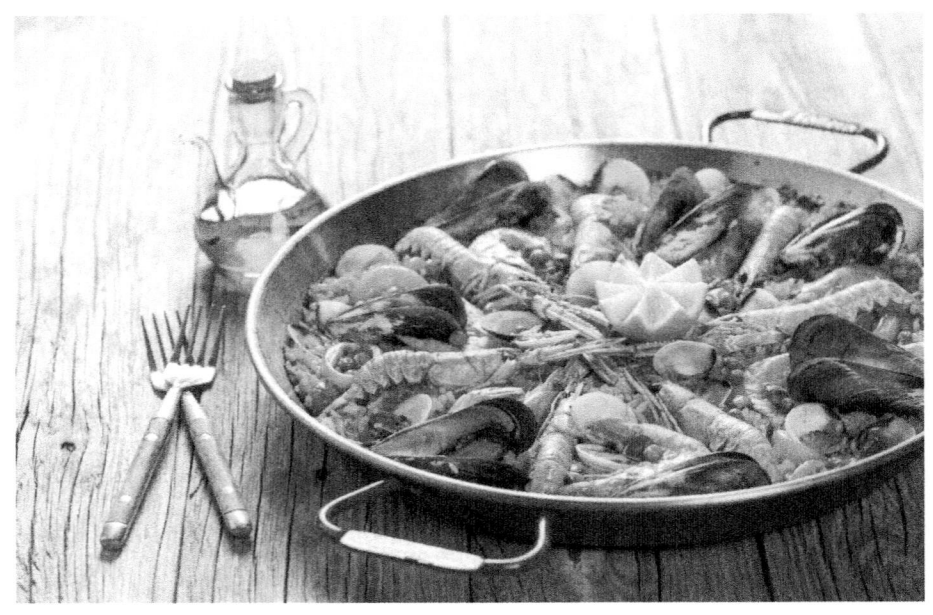

There are many reasons to eat the Mediterranean diet. Rather than a set of diet rules that are hard to remember, this diet focuses on just a few basic changes in lifestyle that are maintainable for the rest of your life. It is about making sure that you get enough physical activity while eating foods that you will truly enjoy. In return, you will enjoy living a fuller life that is free from many chronic health issues.

The first thing that you need to do is eat plenty of fish every week. Eating fish and other seafood is a great way to get Omega 3 fats that are very healthy for you. Had you lived a long time ago, a snake-oil salesman could have made a fortune selling omega 3 fats, but he would have no need to lie. These fats cannot be made by the body, so it is essential to eat them at least two or three times a week. They help to lower the cholesterol level in the body, so you will stand less of a chance of having heart problems. Also helping, eating fish helps to lower the level of triglycerides in the body by at least 30 percent. Scientists also believe that eating fish helps to stop arrhythmias that often lead to sudden heart attacks. Eating fish also helps to stop blood clots from forming that can break off and cause damage. Dining on fish also helps to lower blood pressure. Finally, eating fish helps to stop inflammation in the body.

The second thing that you will want to do is incorporate olive oil in your diet in many different ways. Olive oil provides monounsaturated fatty acids that the body uses to even further lower the risk of heart disease.

Eating olive oil helps to lower a person's total cholesterol, especially low-density lipoprotein cholesterol levels. Recent research also shows that eating olive oil helps to control the body's insulin level and helps the body control the level of blood sugar to avoid spikes. Eating olive oil also makes a person feel full sooner and leave the meal feeling more satisfied. Olive oil contains Vitamins E and K that are essential in fighting many chronic diseases. Furthermore, olive oil contains the antioxidant oleocanthal that helps fight inflammation in the body.

When eating the Mediterranean diet, consume a moderate amount of dairy. Particularly important is Greek yogurt, although the diet does recommend that a person severely limit the amount of crème sauces and high-fat cheeses that they eat. Greek yogurt is high in probiotics that helps to promote a healthy digestive system. The calcium, magnesium and potassium found in Greek yogurt helps to lower blood pressure. According to a study published in the American Journal of Clinical Nutrition, eating dairy products helps a person to lose more weight. The calcium, magnesium, phosphorus, potassium and protein in Greek yogurt promotes healthy bones. Even those who are lactose intolerant often find that they can tolerate a little bit of Greek yogurt, because one cup of nonfat plain Greek yogurt contains only four grams of lactose.

The vast majority of foods eaten on the Mediterranean diet are whole fresh foods including local fruits, vegetables, legumes, and nuts. These foods provide the nutrients that a person needs to thrive. Buying locally grown foods helps to ensure that they taste better, because the food is usually picked the same day that it is sold. Most foods that are even produced in the United States are trucked over 1500 miles before they arrive at your grocery store and may have been picked up to a week ahead of time. That's not to mention the shipping time and distance of foods that come from overseas. The longer a food is in storage, the less nutritious it is for you. Small scale local farmers usually offer a larger diversity of crops, because it allows them to enjoy a longer growing season. Local farmers are your friends and neighbors. Therefore, they take food safety even more serious than larger producers who will never meet their customers. There is no middleman, so often buying locally produced foods means you enjoy saving money when you grocery shop. According to the American Farmland Trust, buying local helps to keep your taxes down because farmers usually pay more in taxes than they require in services. A well-managed farm helps to conserve a way of life, the land and wildlife.

The Mediterranean diet avoids anything processed. Processed foods are usually higher in excess sodium, sugar, fats, and artificial additives. Turn over a package of processed food and look at the ingredient's list. You probably really do not want to know where manufacturers get some of those ingredients. For example, gelatin normally comes from animal skin, while castoreum found in many puddings comes from the secretions of beavers. Researchers at the University of California at Los Angeles have shown that it only takes two months of eating a diet of processed foods to lower a person's IQ. Manufacturers use the same security system found at airports to test for metal in the food before they ship it to grocery stores. Many prepackaged lunch kits contain over 80 different ingredients. Instead of eating food that you have no idea what is, the Mediterranean diet avoids all processed foods.

The focus of the Mediterranean diet is on whole grains. There are numerous benefits to eating whole grains One of the main reasons to eat whole grains are that they are much higher in fiber that help reduce bad cholesterol levels, control blood sugar and helps reduce the risk of colon cancer. Eating whole grains also helps the body digest food properly, and the lactic acid helps produce good bacteria in the large intestine. People who eat whole grains on a daily basis are up to 30 percent less likely to have a heart attack, and are 19 percent less likely to suffer from hypertension. Eating whole grain also helps to keep weight in check. Whole grains are very effective at fighting belly fat. Eating whole grains also helps you to feel full.

Processed sugar is eliminated from the Mediterranean diet. Each person in the United States each an average of 130 pounds of sugar each year. Sugar has been shown to have major detrimental effects on the body's immune system. The body's liver turns unused sugar into fat.

Consuming too much sugar can set one up to travel down the road to diabetes. Sugar can contribute to the formation of cancer. Research has shown that eating a diet high in sugar actually causes a person to feel hungrier. Eating a large amount of sugar causes a dopamine release in the brain. In other words, the body becomes addicted to wanting the sugar. New evidence suggests that consuming a diet high in sugar raises cholesterol, leading to heart attacks, even more than saturated fat.

People on the Mediterranean diet enjoy a glass or two of red wine every day, usually with a meal. Of course, drinking is a personal choice, but for those who choose to drink, drinking red wine has many health benefits. Many red wines contain melatonin that helps to regulate the body's clock so that you get a good night's sleep. Research has shown that the resveratrol compound found in most red wines increases a person's longevity, along with helping to stop Alzheimer's and dementia. Resveratrol has also been shown to lower cholesterol levels and to reduce inflammation. The resveratrol and other antioxidants also helps to keep the heart healthy. According to researchers at the University of Santiago de Compostela in Spain found that drinking just one glass a day reduced the rate of lung disease by 13 percent, while other researchers found that it reduced the chance of prostate cancer by 50 percent. The same researchers in Spain found that people who drank a glass of red wine each day had 44 percent less colds than people who abstained.

While the Mediterranean diet does not totally eliminate red meat, it does suggest that you eat it in extreme moderation. Instead, focus on eating fish along with white meats like chicken and turkey. Eating white meat is a much leaner choice of the protein that your body needs. The protein in white meat helps to prevent bone loss which can start much earlier than you think. White meat generally contains fewer calories. Eating white meat is a natural anti-depressant, because it raises the serotonin levels in your brain. Furthermore, eating white meat helps to control the homocysteine levels in the bloodstream which can lead to heart diseases. White meat is a wonderful source of phosphorous that is needed for strong bones and teeth, as well as to keep the central nervous system functioning properly. The selenium and Vitamin B6 found in white meat helps the body's metabolism and makes sure that you have plenty of energy to get through your day.

The Mediterranean diet also focuses on doing physical activities. Choose a favorite activity and do it every day.

THE MEDITERRANEAN DIET PYRAMID

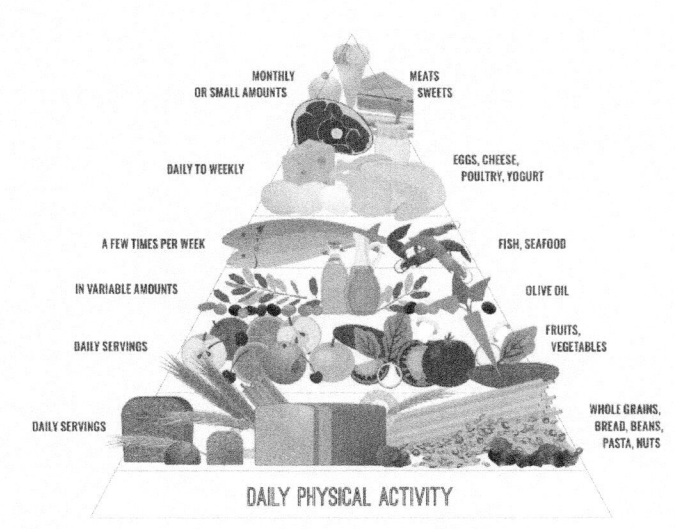

MONTHLY OR SMALL AMOUNTS

MEATS SWEETS

DAILY TO WEEKLY

EGGS, CHEESE, POULTRY, YOGURT

A FEW TIMES PER WEEK

FISH, SEAFOOD

IN VARIABLE AMOUNTS

OLIVE OIL

DAILY SERVINGS

FRUITS, VEGETABLES

DAILY SERVINGS

WHOLE GRAINS, BREAD, BEANS, PASTA, NUTS

DAILY PHYSICAL ACTIVITY

MEDITERRANEAN DIET

The Mediterranean diet is in its nature a Hear-Healthy diet, it's not a "diet" In the strict way of the word, but more of a lifestyle approach to food and eating. As you know now, it's inspired in the Mediterranean countries such as Greece, Spain and Italy, where a big percentage of people don't suffer so much overweight and other forms of disease that are provoked by bad food like in other countries where the basis of food is different.

To better understand the different types of food the Mediterranean Diet is comprised from, and also to make things easier for you when deciding what to eat and what not to eat, there is a very simple "pyramid" that will help you determine if you are in deed applying a Mediterranean Diet approach to your meals.

As you can see, in this diet you have a good amount of ingredients that will make it easy and even enjoyable when doing it. You can even eat sweets as long as you eat them sparingly. Carbohydrates such as whole grains, pasta and bread are actually a very important component of the diet, together with fruits and vegetables.

Take this pyramid when designing your meal plan and always use creativity to make it interesting and delicious for you.

The great thing about the Mediterranean diet is that on top of help you lose weight, it will reduce the risks of hear disease. Since this diet is associated with a lower level of oxidized low-density lipoprotein (LDL) cholesterol, which is the more commonly known as "bad cholesterol" which is the one that have a higher chance of build up deposits in your arteries, which could potentially cause heart disease disorders.

Many studies have shown that following a Mediterranean diet was associated with a much-reduced risk of cardiovascular mortality as well as overall mortality. So, now you know, if you want to increase and enjoy your life, the Mediterranean Diet is a great way to do it.

Those studies have shown also a myriad of benefits also from this diet, such as a reduced incidence of cancer, Parkinson, Alzheimer and even breast cancer, when the diet is supplemented with extra virgin oil and nuts.

Now you should take a second look at the pyramid and see the base of it and read carefully what's written there, yes "Daily Physical Activity". That part is crucial to keep your metabolism running the right way and really helps you to enjoy the Mediterranean lifestyle and lose weight. It doesn't mean that you have to be 5 hours a day at the gym or run a

Marathon, it simply mean that you need to take the time to EVERYDAY do some physical activity, at least 30 minutes. Such as: walking, swimming, running, trekking etc.

So to recap let's make a quick overview of the Key Components you'll need to include in the Mediterranean Diet:

You should eat PRIMARILY plant-based foods (fruits, vegetables, whole grains, legumes and nuts)

Replace butter or other fat you use for cooking with healthy fats such as olive oil or even canola oil

Use more herbs and spices and less salt to flavor your food

Eat red meat only a few times a month

Eat fish and poultry at least twice a week

Drink red wine with moderation

Get plenty of exercise

Enjoy your meals with family and friends

PREPARE YOUR KITCHEN TO COOK EASY AND QUICK

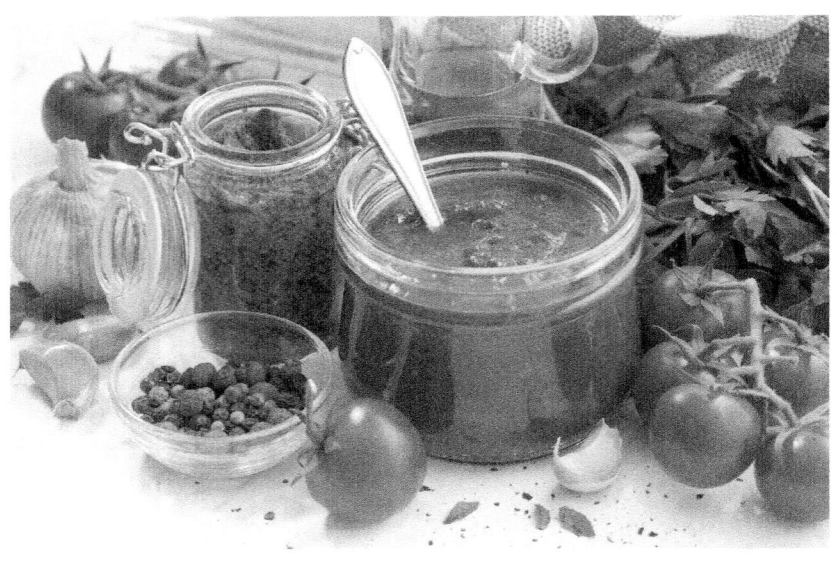

There are several simple steps that you can take in the kitchen to ensure that you are more apt to stay on your diet. Of course, since you get so much food to eat on the Mediterranean diet that it is easy for many people to embrace this new lifestyle, especially when you will soon be feeling so much healthier.

The first step is to empty your refrigerator of all the unhealthy foods. If the rest of your family has not decided to join you in your new lifestyle yet, then it makes it a little harder. Make sure to put a large pitcher of flavored water near the front of the refrigerator and prepare vegetables in snack size plastic bags so that they are easy to grab. Hide as much of the snack food at the back of the refrigerator as possible, and you may soon discover that the rest of your family is eating healthier too.

If you find that it is impossible to remove all the snack food from your house, because of other family members, then also divide these foods into small snack-size packages and hide them as far back in the pantry as possible. Put healthy snacks that you enjoy in front of them, so that they are much easier to grab.

A great tip is to place a large bowl of fruit on the counter where you can easily grab it on your way out the door. This helps ensure that you will not be tempted to stop for a quick bite at the fast food restaurant or grab a candy bar at a convenience store. If you often find that you must eat on the bus or in the car, then make sure to carry packages of nuts and seeds with you, but watch the sodium level.

Keeping a constant shopping list also helps to ensure that you buy the right types of food. Since you will be eating whole foods, you will find that you can cut your shopping time in half, because you will be shopping around the outside of the store and skipping all the processed foods in the middle. Therefore, make sure that you keep a list in your kitchen where you can easily access it as you cook.

Many people find that a great place to keep the list is on the front of the refrigerator, but make sure it is not the only thing found there. Copy some photos of happy times and put them on the front of the fridge. Many people find that keeping photos of family members on the front of the fridge is also a great way to stay motivated by reminding themselves that they want to stay around for those people.

Rather you eat at a designated space in the kitchen or in another room, it is important that you have a designated space that you use only for that purpose. Additionally, make that a happy place where your family will want to linger. On a regular basis, get out the cloth napkins and the tablecloth and make special meals that your family will remember. Additionally, think about incorporating special centerpieces that celebrate holidays or other special occasions.

There are so many different ways that you can spice up the foods that you prepare on the Mediterranean diet. Herbs grow abundantly in the Mediterranean area and they are a great way to increase the flavor of foods. One favorite spice of many people on this diet is oregano which has grown wild in the Mediterranean region for centuries. It is well known for its antioxidant levels. Thyme, fenugreek, capers, cumin, coriander and marjoram are also popular spices included in this diet that have strong antioxidant properties. Additionally, citrus juices are also a popular healthy way to season foods.

As soon as you finish with a meal, take the time to clean up the kitchen properly. That way it will be ready to prepare the next meal. Putting this off just means that you will have to do it later and that often means that it is harder to do as food becomes stuck.

If your kitchen has become full of junk, then eliminate the clutter. Scientists know that working in a clutter-free workspace makes a person happier. Additionally, the clutter makes it hard to be creative as you cook.

Much of the food on the Mediterranean diet is grilled. Therefore, a great addition to the kitchen is a grill. Shoppers find that grills come in three different styles; panini, countertop, and on the range. Panini grills allow users to cook both sides of food at one time. They are most useful, however, for cooking sandwiches and you may not be eating many on the Mediterranean diet. Countertop grills are very similar to outside grills except that they plug into electricity. You can cook almost anything on a countertop grill that you would grill outside including many types of fish and vegetables. Range grills sit on top of the range and use the burners as the heat source. Again, they are useful for cooking many types of food.

The user needs to decide which type of grill is right for them. If the user has the counter space, then many people find that these are most convenient, because it leaves the burners free for other purposes. When buying a countertop grill, look for one that can easily be cleaned. The thicker the cooking surface, the more evenly the grill will cook. These grills generate very little smoke.

Those without the room to spare find that range grills are the perfect solution because it allows them to keep their counter space free for other purposes. They are not designed to be used, however, on glass top stoves. Some of these models can generate a lot of smoke so they are often best used under a cooking hood. If the unit is made with grates, then look for aluminum grates that are lined with porcelain as they are easier to clean and the food will not stick.

Many people enjoy a countertop grill with an aroma scenter. This compartment allows the cook to fill the area with herbs and spices that are infused into the food as it cooks. If the cook enjoys smoke aroma, some even have compartments large enough to put a small handful of wood chips. Another useful component is non-skid feet because this allows the grill to be gently bumped without moving. Look for a grill that has a removable grill top because they are easier to clean.

Before buying a grill consider how many square inches of cooking space is available. Generally, 72 square inches is enough room to prepare three portions of food. If you will be cooking for more people, then you will need a larger unit.

The more metal or silicone is on the grill, generally, the longer it will last. Many of these grills have plastic handles or legs that are known to break off rather easily. An indicator light is a great feature because it lets the cook know when the grill's surface has reached the desired temperature.

When purchasing a grill for the stovetop, look for one that has a cover. This allows the cook to cover the food and helps to control the loss of moisture in the food. Measure the range grill carefully before making a purchase. A convenient feature is that many cover two burners which allows the cook to move food to the center that is cooler while other food is finishing cooking.

There are many ways that you can prepare your kitchen for your new Mediterrean diet. It all starts with removing or hiding unhealthy choices and then making it very easy to get to the foods that you want to eat. A clean kitchen is also a great place to start, as it will keep your creative juices flowing. Additionally, think about getting an indoor grill that allows you to cook either on the countertop or range.

MEDITERRANEAN DIET RECIPES FOR BREAKFAST

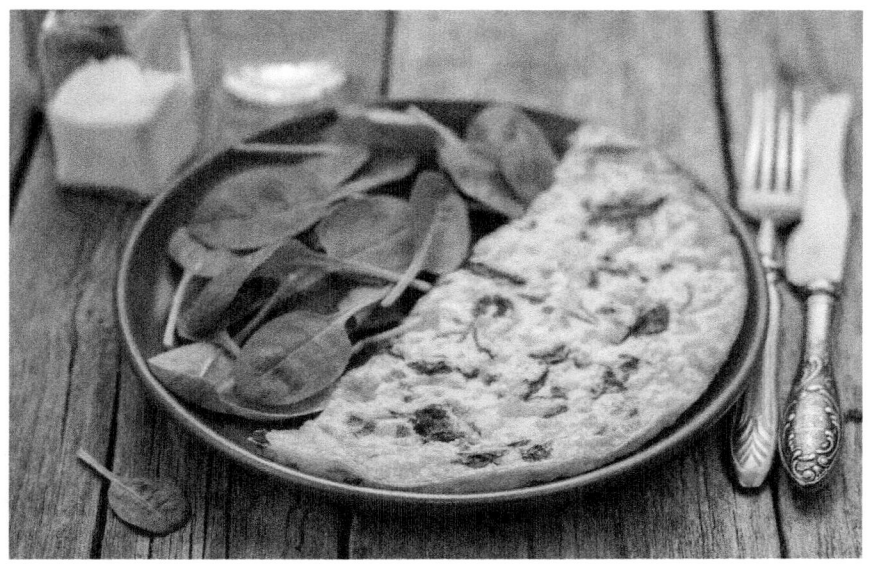

Eating a great breakfast is an awesome way to start every day. You can find many quick recipes that are perfect for that day when everyone is on the fly which is typical of the region where the main meal of the day is usually lunch. Just like in the United States, weekends often include a leisurely breakfast where people linger over their meals. Here are five recipes to get you started.

Potato and Chickpea Hash

Ingredients

4 cups frozen shredded hash brown potatoes

1 small bunch baby spinach

1 small white onion

1 zucchini

1 15 ounce can chickpeas

1 tablespoon fresh ginger

1 tablespoon curry powder

1/2 teaspoon salt

1/4 cup extra-virgin olive oil

4 large eggs

Instructions:

1.Tear baby spinach into bite size pieces to make two cups.

2. Chop onion

3. Chop one zucchini to make one cup

4. Rinse the chickpeas and put in a small bowl.

5. Combine potatoes, spinach, onion, curry powder and salt in a large bowl.

6. Grate curry and add it. Stir until well combined.

7. Heat olive oil over medium-high heat.

8. Add the potato mixture to the skillet and press into a thin layer.

9. Cook for about four minutes until golden brown.

10. Fold in the zucchini and chickpeas. Breaking up any chunks until just combined.

11. Using a large wooden spoon, carve out four-inch wells in the mixture.

12. Break one egg into each well.

13. Cover and cook about four minutes until eggs are soft set.

Whole Wheat Pancakes

Ingredients

1 cup old-fashioned oats

1/2 cup whole-wheat flour

2 tablespoons flax seeds

1 teaspoon baking soda

1/4 teaspoon salt

2 cups plain Greek yogurt

2 large eggs

2 tablespoons honey

2 1/2 tablespoons olive oil

Instructions:

1.Combine oats, whole-wheat flour, flax seeds, baking soda and salt in a blender.

2. Pulse for 30 seconds.

3. Add Greek yogurt, eggs, honey and two tablespoons olive oil.

4. Blend until smooth.

5. Let mixture stand 15 minutes to thicken.

6. Heat non-stick skillet over medium heat.

7. Brush skillet with remaining olive oil.

8. Pour 1/4 cupful of batter onto skillet. Cook until bottom is golden brown.

9. Flip pancake over and finish cooking.

Frittata

Ingredients

1 small white onion

1/2 cup onion-and-garlic croutons

8 eggs

2 cloves garlic, minced

3 tablespoons olive oil

1/4 cup half-and-half

2 ounces feta cheese

1/2 cup chopped bottled roasted red sweet peppers

1/2 cup sliced pitted ripe olives

1/4 cup fresh basil

1/8 teaspoon ground black pepper

2 tablespoons finely shredded Parmesan cheese

Instructions:

1.Chop the onion.

2. In a medium bowl, beat the eggs

3. Crush the croutons in another small bowl.

4. Preheat broiler.

5. In a broiler proof pan, mince the garlic and cook it and the onion in two tablespoons oil until translucent.

6. Add the cream to the eggs and whisk.

7. Add feta cheese, roasted sweet pepper, olives (if desired), basil, and black pepper to the egg mixture. Stir until well combined.

8. Pour egg mixture over onion mixture.

9. Cook mixture until eggs are soft set.

10. In a separate bowl, combine crushed croutons, Parmesan cheese, and the remaining tablespoon of oil.

11. Sprinkle mixture over egg mixture.

12. Put in broiler and broil for three minutes.

Omelet

1 medium tomato

1 capsicum

1/4 cup pitted Kalamata olives

2 cloves garlic

2 green onions

1 tablespoon. extra virgin olive oil

1tablespoon. lemon juice

1 tablespoon fresh chopped parsley

2 tablespoons skimmed milk

4 eggs

1 teaspoon chives

1 teaspoon oregano

1 teaspoon basil

2 ounces feta cheese

Instructions

1. Dice tomato and green onion

2. In a small bowl, combine tomatoes, capsicum, olives, garlic, green onions, olive oil, lemon juice and parsley.

3. In a small bowl, whisk together eggs, milk, chives, oregano, basil and feta cheese.

4. Sir tomato mixture into egg mixture.

5. Cook in a non-stick skillet for two minutes.

6. Divide the mixture into two. Fold each half over onto its self. Then, flip each half over.

7. Cover skillet and cool one more minutes.

Mexican Scramble

1/4 cup olive oil

3 jalapeños

1 small yellow onion

5 cloves garlic

1 teaspoon ground cumin

1 tablespoon paprika

1 28-ounce can whole peeled tomatoes, undrained

1/8 teaspoon Kosher salt, to taste

6 eggs

1/2 cup feta cheese,

1 tablespoon chopped parsley

Instructions:

1. Slice jalapenos down the middle. Remove seeds. Chop.

2. Dice onion

3. Slice garlic extremely thin.

4. Heat oil in a 12-inch skillet until hot.

5. Add onions and peppers. Cook until onion starts to turn brown.

6. Add cumin, paprika and garlic. Cook until garlic is soft.

7. Crush tomatoes and add them to the skillet. Do not drain.

8. Add 1/2 cup water.

9. Reduce heat and simmer until mixture thickens. This will take about 15 minutes.

10. Add eggs over top. Do not stir.

11. Cook until eggs are desired doneness.

MEDITERRANEAN DIET RECIPES FOR LUNCH

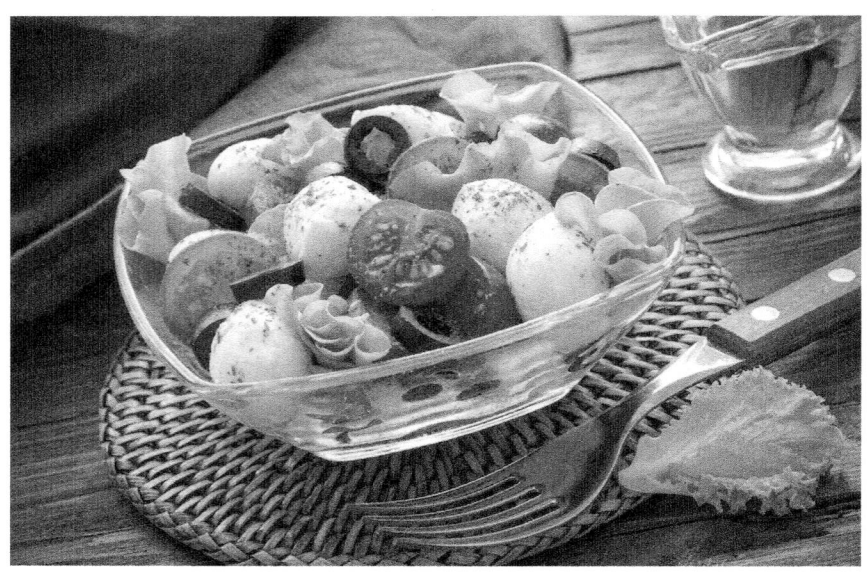

It is so easy to prepare a great lunch on the go when you are eating the Mediterranean diet. In addition to getting to stay with your new lifestyle, you get to enjoy the savings from not eating out. Here are five recipes to get you started.

Mediterranean Tuna Salad

Ingredients

12 ounces canned tuna

1/4 cup mayonnaise

1/4 cup pitted ripe olives

1/4 cup bottled roasted red peppers

2 green onions

1 tablespoon small capers

6 slices whole wheat bread

Instructions:

1.Drain tuna and put in a bowl. Flake with a fork.

2. Add mayonnaise to tuna and stir until well combined.

3. Chop olives and add to the mixture.

4. Drain and chop the red peppers. Add to the mixture.

5. Rinse and drain the capers. Add them to the mixture.

6. Chop the green onions and add them.

7. Lay out the bread and divide the mixture between the slices.

Stuffed Tomatoes

Ingredients:

2 large tomatoes

1/2 cup packaged garlic croutons

1/4 cup (1 ounce) crumbled goat cheese

1/4 cup sliced pitted kalamata olives

2 tablespoons reduced-fat vinaigrette or Italian salad dressing

2 tablespoons chopped fresh thyme or basil

Instructions:

1.Wash tomatoes and slice in half. Remove seeds and pulp. Save the pulp in a medium mixing bowl.

2. Place hollowed out tomatoes on a paper towel. Let drain for five minutes.

3. Add remaining ingredients to tomato pulp. Chop and stir until well combined.

4. Using a spoon, mound mixture into hollowed out tomatoes.

5. Place tomatoes on baking sheet.

6. Put under broiler for five minutes.

Garbanzo Chicken Salad

Ingredients

1 cooked chicken breast

1 (15-ounce) can chickpeas

1 small cucumber

4 green onions

1 bunch basil

1/2 cup plain fat-free yogurt

2 garlic cloves

1/4 teaspoon salt

2 cups prepackaged baby spinach leaves

1/3 cup (1.3 ounces) feta cheese with cracked pepper, crumbled

4 lemon wedges

Instructions:

1.Chop cucumber fine.

2. Chop green onions.

3. Chop basil.

4. Chop chicken breast into bite size pieces.

5. Combine chicken, cucumber, green onions, basil, and baby spinach, yogurt and minced garlic. Mix until well combined.

6. Add chickpeas and mix again.

7. Distribute feta cheese over top of salad.

8. Lay lemon wedges on salad.

Pita Bake

6 ounce tub sun-dried tomato pesto

6 6 inch whole wheat pita breads

2 Roma tomatoes

1 bunch spinach

4 fresh mushrooms

1/2 cup crumbled feta cheese

2 tablespoons grated Parmesan cheese

1 tablespoon olive oil

1/8 teaspoon pepper

Instructions:

1.Preheat oven to 350 degrees.

2. Chop Roma tomatoes

3. Tear spinach into bite-size pieces

4. Spread pesto on one side of pita bread.

5. Top pesto with remaining ingredients.

6. Bake pitas on baking sheet. Bake for 15 minutes.

Quinoa Salad

Ingredients

2 cubes chicken bouillon

1 clove garlic

1 cup uncooked quinoa

2 large cooked chicken breasts

1 large red onion

1 large green bell pepper

1/2 cup chopped kalamata olives

1/2 cup crumbled feta cheese

1/4 cup fresh parsley

1/4 cup fresh chives

1/2 teaspoon salt

2/3 cup fresh lemon juice

1 tablespoon balsamic vinegar

1/4 cup olive oil

Instructions:

1.Cut chicken breast into bite sized pieces.

2. Dice onion and bell pepper.

3. Mince garlic and put in saucepan with bouillon cubes and water.
Bring to a boil.

4. Stir in quinoa, reduce heat to medium, and cover pan.

5. Cook until all water is absorbed which will take about 15 minutes.

6. Place the quinoa in a large bowl.

7. Stir in chicken, onion, bell pepper, olives, feta cheese, parsley, chives
and salt. Mix until well combined.

8. Drizzle lemon juice, balsamic vinegar and olive oil over top. Stirring to
combine well.

9. Refrigerate overnight.

MEDITERRANEAN DIET RECIPES FOR DINNER

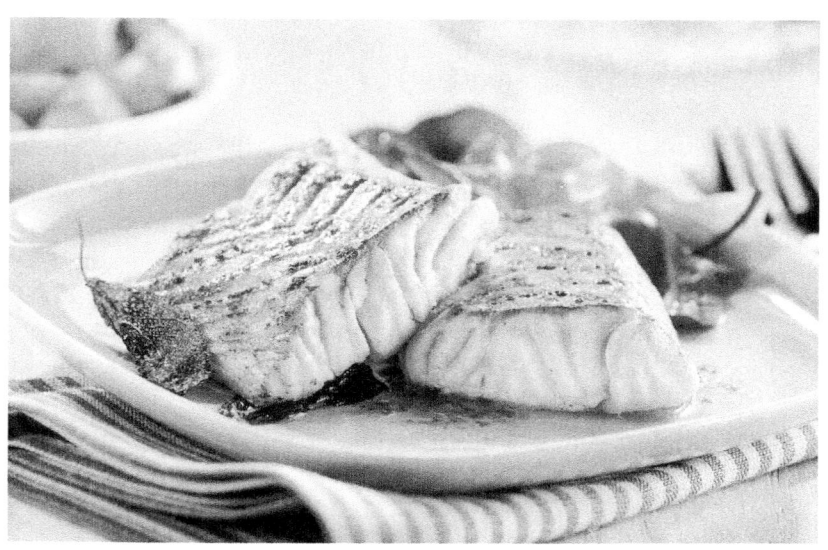

With a multitude of options available for dinner, the Mediterranean diet is easy to prepare and follow when dinner rolls around. Here are some of the favorite options.

Garlic Lime Grilled Chicken

Ingredients

6 ounces chicken breast

2 minced garlic cloves

1 tsp salt

1 tsp pepper

3 tsp lime juice

Instructions

1. In a container large enough for your chicken mix your ingredients to make your marinade.

2. Cover both sides of your chicken with a brush. Leave in your refrigerator for at least a hour.

3. You can take this time to cut up a onion, some tomatoes and a cucumber if you'd like your chicken with salad which is a great choice.

4. Turn on your grill and get it nice and hot.

5. Throw on your chicken cooking for six minutes before flipping over. Cook until there's no pink inside.

6. When you have about a minute left, toss a cup and a half of your choice of salad (I like spinach) with olive oil to taste, top with your onions, tomatoes and cucumber, plate your chicken and dinner is ready.

7. Enjoy with a glass of heart healthy red wine!

Mediterranean Mozzarella Baked Salmon

Ingredients

5oz Salmon Filet

2 tsp olive oil

3 tsp lemon juice

1 tsp soy sauce

2 oz mozzarella cheese

Salt and pepper

One of my favourite Mediterranean Diet dinner options, easy to prepare, healthy and tastes amazing!

Instructions

1. Combine the olive oil, lemon juice and soy sauce and marinate your salmon for 30 minutes.

2. Set your oven to 350 degrees. Spray a oven tray with no stick spray and place your salmon on it and go into the oven.

3. Check in 15 minutes to see if salmon has reached your desired temperature. I prefer mine medium rare.

4. Pull out when ready, sprinkle with salt and pepper to taste. Top with 2 oz mozzarella cheese drizzle with balsamic vinegar and you're ready to go! Works well with lots of sides.

Grilled Swordfish with Zucchini and Squash pasta

Ingredients

5 oz Swordfish

one small zucchini and one small yellow squash

a small onion

2 tsp olive oil

1 tsp lemon

salt and pepper

4 oz of angel hair pasta

Instructions

1. Cut your zucchini and squash into small half moons and dice as much onion as you'd like.

2. Boil water for your pasta.

3. Rub the swordfish with oil and lemon and toss on grill. It cooks very quickly so pay attention about 3 minutes on each side.

4. Sauté your veggies in a pan while grilling fish.

5. Throw pasta in water. Drain pasta when 3/4's done and toss in olive oil with veggies.

6. Place in bowl and top with sword fish. Sprinkle with salt and pepper to taste - also a bit of oregano adds a nice touch! Sounds good doesn't it?

Hope you enjoy these Mediterranean Diet dinner options! Do you have any favorites I missed?

you have any favorites I missed?

FINAL THOUGHTS

The Mediterranean style food is delicious and feels less like a diet than many of the health food choices available. If you haven't heard already, the latest research shows that a diet based on Mediterranean style cooking can reduce the risk of heart disease, stroke and heart attack by as much as thirty percent.

After conducting a study that lasted five years, researchers found that a diet consisting of foods such as olive oil, nuts, produce and fish was significantly more effective in reducing the risk of chronic conditions like stroke and heart disease than a low fat diet. Researchers believe that the combination of nutrient-rich compounds and healthy fats found in Mediterranean style food is what accounts for the benefits to cardiovascular health that they found in the study.

That's good news for you. Mediterranean style food will keep you healthy and, as many others have found, it will help you lose weight as well. It's light on the wallet too. Many of the ingredients such as veggies, nuts, beans, fish and olive oil are inexpensive when compared to other dietary foods. If you have been living on protein bars, juice cleansers, and other supplemental food, then you're in for a surprise when you see how much cheaper Mediterranean style food can be. And, it's delicious too!

Following a Mediterranean diet is simple enough. Just add the following components to your daily routine.

- Eat mainly plant-based food. This includes fruit, vegetables, legumes, whole grains and nuts.

- Drink a glass of red wine with dinner. No more than seven glasses a week.

- Replace butter with extra-virgin olive oil or another source of healthy fats.

- Avoid salt. Use herbs and spices to flavor your food.

- Eat more fish and poultry. You should have these at least twice a week but more often is fine.

- Limit your red meat consumption. Red meat is still important, but try to eat it no more than a few times per month.

This is a diet that you can follow pretty easily. You can find extra-virgin olive oil in just about every super market along with fresh fruit and vegetables. If you can, try to obtain fresh fish from a fish market. For poultry and red meat, visit your local butcher to get the healthiest cuts.

I hope you enjoyed this introductory guide to the Mediterranean Diet and now get out there and start living the lifestyle.

Bonus Book

In The Mediterranean Diet book you have found a good number of strategies to build a healthier style of living and to lose weight by doing it.

However if you want to take a more hands-on approach I'd like to give away for you a book that will help you get there and achieve your objectives faster. Just head to my website at http://dieterspro.com and download your copy now.

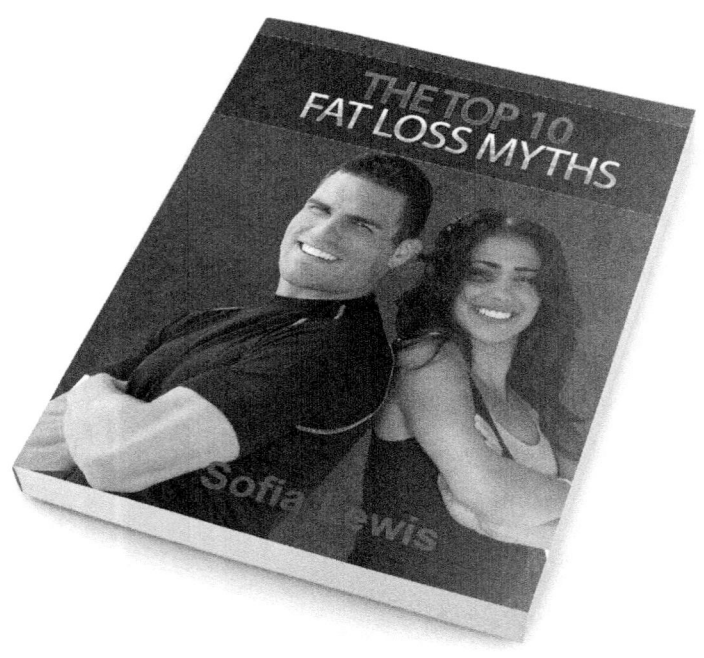

www.DietersPro.com